LUPUS DIET COOKBOOK

Anti-Inflammatory Recipes For Managing Symptoms, Boosting Immunity, And Enhancing Wellness

DR ELIAN GRIFFIN

DISCLAIMER

The nutritional recommendations and recipes in this book are meant solely for informative reasons. They are not meant to replace the counsel, diagnosis, or care of a qualified medical expert. If you have any doubts about a medical condition or dietary requirements, you should always see your physician or another trained healthcare expert.

All reasonable efforts have been taken by the author and publisher to ensure that the information contained in this book is correct as of the date of publication. Recommendations may alter, though, as medical knowledge is always changing. When using any of the recipes or instructions found here, the user assumes all liability and assumes no risk, whether personal or otherwise. People who have certain dietary requirements or medical issues should speak with a healthcare provider for personalized guidance. The given recipes are only ideas; you may need to adjust them to suit your own nutritional needs, tastes, and tolerances.

When you use this book, you agree to release the publisher, the author, and their representatives from any liability for any claims, damages, liabilities, costs, or expenditures resulting from your use of the book.

TABLE OF CONTENTS

ABOUT THE BOOK

Lupus, a chronic autoimmune disease, has a profound impact on daily life, and dietary choices can significantly influence symptoms and overall well-being. It is important to understand how specific foods affect inflammation, energy levels, joint health, and more to improve the quality of life for those who have lupus. The "Lupus Diet Cookbook" is an invaluable resource for anyone navigating the complexities of managing lupus through nutrition.

The management of lupus symptoms is largely dependent on nutrition. A balanced diet customized for lupus patients can help reduce inflammation, and and fatigue, and support overall health. This cookbook offers detailed instructions on how to incorporate foods high in vital nutrients while avoiding triggers that may exacerbate symptoms. The recipes emphasize anti-inflammatory ingredients and support gut health, so they not only support physical wellness but also foster a pleasurable eating experience.

Beginning with an overview of lupus and its nutritional implications, the cookbook explores the causes and symptoms of the disease, emphasizing the role that diet plays in managing symptoms and outlining the essential nutrients needed for optimal health.

It also offers helpful advice on how to assess current dietary practices, set realistic goals, and create customized meal plans, enabling readers to make long-lasting changes that will lead to improved health outcomes.

This cookbook offers a wide range of recipes that are tailored to the dietary requirements of individuals with lupus. From filling and healthy breakfasts to hearty lunches and delectable dinners, every recipe is thoughtfully created with components that support digestive health, enhance joint health, and give long-lasting energy.

Snack and dessert options satisfy cravings without sacrificing health objectives, providing guilt-free treats that fit into a lupus-friendly diet.

Social events and holidays present special difficulties for people with lupus. This cookbook gives readers tips on how to handle these situations and still follow diet rules. It offers holiday menus and festive desserts that put health first so that you can enjoy life to the fullest on all occasions.

Along with practical advice for dining out and reading food labels, the cookbook also tackles common issues and frequently asked questions, such as handling dietary restrictions, navigating food allergies, and understanding potential interactions between food and medication. These resources empower readers to make decisions that support their health goals.

Essentially, the "Lupus Diet Cookbook" is much more than a cookbook; it is an all-encompassing manual for adopting a way of life that regulates lupus symptoms via careful nutrition.

CHAPTER ONE

WHAT IS LUPUS AND HOW DOES IT IMPACT NUTRITION

Lupus is an autoimmune disease in which the immune system attacks healthy tissues and organs, causing inflammation, pain, and damage throughout the body, including the joints, skin, kidneys, heart, and even the brain. For those who have lupus, managing symptoms often entails medication, lifestyle modifications, and dietary changes to support overall health and reduce inflammation.

Understanding these dietary principles enables individuals with lupus to make informed choices that promote wellness and effectively manage symptoms. Dietary factors are important in managing lupus symptoms because certain foods can either trigger or help alleviate inflammation. Common triggers include foods high in sugars, processed ingredients, and saturated fats.

On the other hand, a diet rich in antioxidants, omega-3 fatty acids, and nutrients like vitamins D and B can help reduce inflammation and support immune function.

Understanding the impact of lupus on diet and making thoughtful dietary choices can help individuals better manage their condition and improve their quality of life. Adopting a balanced approach that includes plenty of fresh fruits and vegetables, lean proteins, and whole grains is more important than simply avoiding triggers when it comes to adjusting to a lupus-friendly diet. It also helps maintain a healthy weight and reduces inflammation.

NUTRITION IS KEY TO MANAGING SYMPTOMS OF LUPUS

A well-balanced diet can help reduce inflammation, boost energy, support immune function, and improve overall well-being for people living with lupus. By focusing on nutrient-dense foods and avoiding triggers that exacerbate symptoms, people can greatly improve their quality of life and manage the disease more effectively. Nutrition is crucial in managing lupus symptoms and overall health.

Antioxidant-rich foods like berries, spinach, and nuts can help combat oxidative stress and support immune function. Adequate intake of vitamin D and B complex vitamins is also crucial for maintaining bone health and supporting energy levels, which can be affected by lupus-related fatigue. Key nutrients like omega-3 fatty acids found in fish like salmon and flaxseeds can help reduce inflammation and alleviate joint pain associated with lupus.

Focusing on nutrient density and culinary creativity, this cookbook empowers people with lupus to take charge of their health through mindful eating and enjoyable cooking experiences. It does this by offering enticing and nutritious recipes that are geared toward supporting overall health and symptom management. By incorporating these recipes into daily meals, people can proactively manage their condition and enjoy flavorful dishes that promote wellness.

With a focus on ingredients that promote anti-inflammatory effects and overall wellness, this cookbook offers a variety of delectable recipes that are also specifically tailored to support lupus management. The purpose of the lupus diet cookbook is to be a useful resource for individuals looking to manage their condition through diet.

This cookbook offers a variety of recipes that emphasize flavor and nutrient density without sacrificing health benefits. From salads full of antioxidants to hearty soups full of vegetables and lean proteins, each dish is designed to support immune function and nourish the body. It also includes meal planning ideas and substitution suggestions to make it easier for people to make these recipes a regular part of their diets.

In addition to recipes, this cookbook is an instructional resource that sheds light on the relationship between diet and lupus symptoms.

CHAPTER TWO

COMPREHENDING DIET AND LUPUS

AN OVERVIEW OF THE CAUSES AND SYMPTOMS OF LUPUS

Although the exact cause of lupus is unknown, it is thought to result from a combination of genetic, environmental, and hormonal factors. Certain triggers, like infections, sunlight exposure, and stress, can exacerbate symptoms. Additionally, hormonal imbalances, particularly in women, are thought to play a significant role, as lupus is more common in females, especially those of childbearing age. Lupus is a chronic autoimmune disease where the body's immune system mistakenly attacks healthy tissues, leading to inflammation and damage in various body parts, including the skin, joints, kidneys, and other organs.

No one test can diagnose lupus; instead, a combination of physical examinations, blood tests, and urine tests are usually used.

The symptoms of lupus are varied and can differ significantly from person to person. Common signs include fatigue, joint pain, swelling, and skin rashes, especially a rash that spreads across the nose and cheeks.

Other symptoms may include fever, hair loss, and sensitivity to sunlight. In severe cases, lupus can affect vital organs like the heart, lungs, and kidneys, which can result in complications like kidney failure, heart disease, or lung issues.

Living with lupus means managing symptoms and avoiding flare-ups. Patients and healthcare providers collaborate to customize treatments, which may involve corticosteroids, immunosuppressants, and nonsteroidal anti-inflammatory drugs (NSAIDs).

Lifestyle modifications, such as eating a balanced diet, controlling stress, and avoiding known triggers, are essential for maintaining general health. Regular follow-up and modifications to treatment regimens enable people with lupus to lead active, fulfilling lives despite the obstacles the disease presents.

HOW FOOD AFFECTS SYMPTOMS OF LUPUS

A healthy diet is essential for controlling the symptoms of lupus because certain foods can either make the condition worse or make it better. Anti-inflammatory foods, like whole grains, fatty fish, and fruits and vegetables, can help lower inflammation and lessen the frequency and intensity of flare-ups. For instance, omega-3 fatty acids, which are found in fish like salmon and mackerel, can lower inflammation and promote heart health.

Antioxidants, which are found in fruits and vegetables like spinach and berries, can shield cells from oxidative stress, which is especially helpful for lupus patients.

On the other hand, certain foods can exacerbate inflammation and exacerbate the symptoms of lupus. Processed foods high in sugars and saturated fats, along with those containing additives and preservatives, can exacerbate inflammation and have a detrimental effect on general health. Dairy products and gluten-containing grains are frequently associated with inflammation in some lupus patients, so cutting back on their intake may help manage symptoms. Additionally, patients are advised to avoid alcohol and caffeine as they can impair the effectiveness of medication and exacerbate kidney health issues.

Incorporating foods high in fiber, like legumes, whole grains, and vegetables, can help maintain a healthy gut microbiome, which is essential for immune function. It's also important to stay hydrated by drinking plenty of water and herbal teas, as these can also help flush out toxins and reduce inflammation.

For a balanced approach, many lupus patients find it beneficial to work with a nutritionist or dietitian who can help tailor a diet plan that meets their specific health needs and lifestyle.

CRUCIAL DIETARY REQUIREMENTS FOR PATIENTS WITH LUPUS

For those who have lupus, maintaining sufficient intake of vital nutrients is critical to both managing the disease and improving overall well-being. Protein is required for tissue repair and muscle mass maintenance, so eating lean meats, beans, and legumes is advised. Omega-3 fatty acids, which can be found in walnuts, flaxseed, and fatty fish, are especially helpful because they have anti-inflammatory qualities.

Vitamin D, calcium, and magnesium are vital vitamins and minerals that are necessary for maintaining bone health, which is compromised by the use of steroid medications frequently prescribed for lupus treatment.

It is equally important to focus on electrolyte balance and hydration because dehydration can exacerbate lupus symptoms and kidney problems. You can help maintain fluid balance by drinking lots of water and eating foods high in electrolytes, such as spinach, bananas, and nuts.

You can also protect cells from oxidative damage by including antioxidants, like vitamins C and E, in your diet by including a variety of colorful fruits and vegetables. You can also add green tea, which has anti-inflammatory and antioxidant properties, to your diet.

Furthermore, foods high in selenium, like Brazil nuts, sunflower seeds, and mushrooms, are important because selenium has been shown to help reduce inflammation and support immune function.

A balanced diet that includes these essential nutrients can significantly improve the quality of life for lupus patients, helping them manage their symptoms and maintain better overall health.

Probiotics and probiotics also support gut health, which is crucial for a strong immune system. Yogurt, kefir, and fermented foods like sauerkraut can enhance gut flora diversity.

Selecting foods that boost immune function and lower inflammation is crucial when managing lupus through diet. Antioxidants, omega-3 fatty acids, and fiber-rich foods are good choices for a lupus-friendly diet. Berries, leafy greens, and cruciferous vegetables, like broccoli and cauliflower, are great options because they are high in vitamins and minerals that help fight inflammation. Fatty fish, like salmon, sardines, and mackerel, offer omega-3 fatty acids that can help reduce joint pain and stiffness. Whole grains, nuts, and seeds are also beneficial because they offer necessary nutrients and promote digestive health.

On the other hand, some foods can exacerbate lupus symptoms and cause inflammation, so it's important to avoid or limit them. Refined foods, processed foods high in sugars, dairy products, and grains containing gluten, such as wheat, barley, and rye, should be avoided as they can stress the immune system and cause inflammation.

High-sodium foods and those with artificial additives and preservatives should also be avoided as they can cause kidney problems and fluid retention.

A lupus patient's diet can be tailored to support their health, reduce inflammation, and improve their quality of life by focusing on whole, minimally processed foods. Whole foods, such as citrus fruits, nuts, and seeds, are rich in vitamins C and E, which can help the body fight inflammation. Spices, such as ginger and turmeric, are excellent for their anti-inflammatory properties and can be easily added to dishes for flavor and health benefits.

ADVANTAGES OF EATING A DIET FRIENDLY TO LUPUS

A lupus-friendly diet can be very beneficial to the quality of life of people who have the disease. Anti-inflammatory foods, like fruits, vegetables, whole grains, and fatty fish, help lower inflammation and lessen the frequency and intensity of flare-ups. Eating this way can also increase energy levels, improve mood, strengthen the immune system, and help people manage their daily activities more easily.

Finally, keeping a healthy weight with a balanced diet can lessen the strain on joints and organs, which will improve overall health.

Consuming foods high in antioxidants and omega-3 fatty acids helps protect kidney tissues from damage. Consuming plenty of water and including kidney-friendly foods like berries, leafy greens, and cruciferous vegetables can further safeguard kidney health. Reducing sodium intake and avoiding foods high in additives and preservatives can help manage blood pressure and reduce the risk of kidney damage, which is a significant concern for many lupus patients.

Eating a diet low in these nutrients also supports better kidney function, which is important because lupus can lead to kidney complications.

Maintaining a lupus-friendly diet over time can result in long-term health benefits and an improved quality of life. Patients can experience decreased inflammation, pain, and symptoms by reducing their intake of pro-inflammatory foods and increasing their intake of nutrient-dense options. This dietary approach not only helps manage symptoms but also improves overall well-being, enabling lupus patients to live more actively and comfortably. With the help of healthcare professionals and dietitians, lupus patients can successfully make dietary changes that have a significant impact on their health journey.

CHAPTER THREE

EVALUATING YOUR EXISTING LIFESTYLE AND DIET

To begin a Lupus diet, you must first evaluate your current diet and lifestyle. This entails examining what you usually eat, your eating habits, and how these may affect your general health, especially Lupus symptoms. To start, keep a food diary for a week, recording everything you eat and when. This will assist you in identifying any triggers or patterns that may be affecting your symptoms. You should also evaluate your lifestyle habits, including how much physical activity you do, how you handle stress, and how you sleep, as these also play a major role in managing Lupus.

This assessment phase lays the groundwork for making well-informed dietary changes that support your overall well-being with Lupus. Once you have a clear picture of your current diet and lifestyle, you can then identify areas that may need adjustment.

Look for any foods that seem to exacerbate your symptoms or cause discomfort. It's also important to evaluate your nutrient intake to ensure you're getting adequate vitamins, minerals, and other essential nutrients. Speaking with a registered dietitian who specializes in autoimmune conditions or a healthcare professional can offer insightful advice based on your individual needs and symptoms.

CREATING PRACTICAL OBJECTIVES FOR DIETARY ADJUSTMENTS

The key to a successful lupus diet is setting realistic goals for dietary changes. Based on your assessment, identify specific areas you want to improve on. These goals should be attainable and customized to your unique needs and lifestyle. For example, if you have identified certain foods that trigger inflammation, your goal may be to gradually reduce or eliminate them from your diet. Another goal may be to increase your intake of anti-inflammatory foods that have been shown to benefit lupus sufferers, such as leafy greens, fatty fish rich in omega-3 fatty acids, and vibrant fruits and vegetables.

To avoid feeling overwhelmed, break larger goals into smaller, manageable steps. For example, instead of completely overhauling your diet overnight, focus on making one or two changes each week, like replacing sugary snacks with healthier alternatives or cooking more meals at home using fresh ingredients.

Celebrate each small success along the way, as this positive reinforcement helps maintain motivation and momentum toward achieving your dietary goals. Flexibility and patience are key when setting goals. After all, Rome wasn't built in a day, and neither can dietary changes.

Having a support system can help you stick to your dietary changes. Remember, the key to setting realistic goals is to make gradual, sustainable changes that enhance your quality of life with lupus and are in line with your health priorities.

Finally, share your goals with those closest to you, such as family or friends, so they can offer encouragement and support.

FORMULATING A WELL-BALANCED DIET FOR LUPUS

A balanced lupus diet plan incorporates foods that boost immunity and lower inflammation while making sure you get enough nutrients. You should emphasize eating a range of nutrient-dense foods in your meals, such as lean proteins (fish, chicken, and legumes) that provide essential amino acids for immune system function and muscle repair, and whole grains (quinoa, brown rice, and oats) that provide fiber and B vitamins that are important for energy metabolism and digestive health.

To ensure a wide range of vitamins, minerals, and antioxidants, emphasize the importance of fruits and vegetables. Foods high in antioxidants, such as berries, spinach, sweet potatoes, and bell peppers, can help fight the oxidative stress associated with lupus. You should also think about including healthy fats, such as those found in avocados, olive oil, and nuts, which provide omega-3 fatty acids and are known to have anti-inflammatory properties. Dairy or dairy substitutes fortified with calcium and vitamin D are also vital for maintaining bone health, which is especially important for lupus patients who may be more susceptible to osteoporosis.

Planning your meals and snacks will help you stick to your dietary goals and make healthier choices. You can also keep your meals interesting and flavorful by experimenting with different recipes and cooking techniques. Speaking with a registered dietitian who specializes in autoimmune conditions can also provide personalized guidance and ensure that your diet plan meets your specific nutritional needs while effectively managing your Lupus symptoms.

OVERVIEW OF INGREDIENTS FRIENDLY TO LUPUS

Adding foods that boost immune function and reduce inflammation is the main goal of this introduction to lupus-friendly ingredients. Let's start by getting acquainted with foods that are known to help people with lupus. These include foods high in antioxidants, like berries, dark leafy greens, and vibrant veggies like carrots and beets. Free radical damage can cause inflammation and accelerate the course of the disease in lupus.

Consume lean protein sources like turkey, chicken, fish, tofu, and legumes like lentils and chickpeas. These proteins offer essential amino acids needed to sustain immune system function and maintain muscle mass. Omega-3 fatty acids, which are present in fatty fish like salmon, mackerel, and sardines, as well as in walnuts and flaxseeds, have anti-inflammatory qualities that can help lessen inflammation and symptoms associated with lupus.

Finally, include healthy fats from sources like avocados, olive oil, and nuts, which support cardiovascular health and provide energy.

Whole grains, such as brown rice, quinoa, and whole wheat bread, offer fiber and important nutrients like iron and B vitamins.

Fiber also helps promote digestive health and can aid in managing blood sugar levels and weight, which are important considerations for individuals with Lupus.

ADVICE ON ORGANIZING AND PREPARING MEALS

Maintaining a Lupus-friendly diet that supports your overall health and well-being requires effective meal planning and preparation. To begin, schedule some time each week to plan your meals and snacks. Take into account your schedule and opt for easy-to-prepare recipes, like casseroles, stews, and soups. This will help reduce the stress and fatigue that come with preparing daily meals while guaranteeing you have nutrient-dense options on hand.

Aim for balance and variety in your meal planning; make sure each meal includes a mix of whole grains, lean proteins, fruits, and vegetables to ensure you're getting a variety of nutrients. Batch-cooking larger portions make it easier to portion out meals for the coming week or freeze extras for later use, so you can follow your diet without feeling overwhelmed.

Consider using cooking methods that require less hands-on time, such as slow cookers, instant pots, or sheet pan meals, which can streamline meal preparation while maximizing flavor and nutrition. Label and date containers to easily identify meals and ingredients in your refrigerator or freezer. Invest in high-quality storage containers and meal prep tools to keep your food fresh and organized.

Last but not least, pay attention to how different foods make you feel and modify your meal planning and preparation techniques accordingly. Speaking with a registered dietitian with expertise in lupus can offer tailored advice and assist in creating a meal plan that satisfies your specific nutritional requirements while successfully managing symptoms.

CHAPTER FOUR

MEAL PLANNING: RECIPES FOR BREAKFAST

ENERGIZING AND NUTRITIOUS BREAKFAST IDEAS

With these delicious and nutritious breakfast ideas designed for a lupus-friendly diet, you can start your day with a boost of energy and nutrients. For those who prefer a savory option, make a veggie-packed omelet with bell peppers, spinach, and a sprinkle of turmeric for its anti-inflammatory properties. Serve it with a slice of gluten-free toast topped with avocado for healthy fats and fiber. Start with a hearty smoothie packed with antioxidant-rich berries, spinach, and a scoop of protein powder to support muscle health. Blend with almond milk for a creamy texture and added calcium.

For a heartier option, try overnight oats made with gluten-free oats, almond milk, and a combination of nuts and seeds for extra protein and omega-3s. You can add fresh fruits like bananas or berries for a refreshing twist.

If you're looking for a warming breakfast on chilly mornings, try quinoa porridge cooked in almond milk with a dash of vanilla extract and cinnamon. You can add chopped nuts and dried fruits for sweetness and crunch. This will guarantee a well-balanced start to your day that keeps you feeling full and nourished.

EASY BREAKFAST RECIPES FOR BUSY MORNINGS

For a nutrient-dense, filling breakfast, make a batch of chia seed pudding the night before and let it thicken in the refrigerator. Another option is a Greek yogurt parfait layered with granola and mixed berries, which provides probiotics for gut health and antioxidants to support your immune system. These quick and easy breakfast ideas ensure you start your day right without compromising on nutrition when time is short.

To make a healthy breakfast that you can grab on the go, try making some gluten-free muffins with oats, nuts, and seeds. You can customize these muffins with your favorite ingredients to make them even more convenient.

You can also make a green smoothie with spinach, banana, and almond milk to get a quick boost of vitamins and minerals. If you want to add some extra protein to your smoothie, it can be especially useful on busy mornings when you need sustained energy.

RECIPES PACKED WITH VITAL NUTRIENTS

Make sure that your lupus diet includes this tasty and nutrient-dense avocado toast with smoked salmon and chia seeds. The avocado offers healthy fats and fiber, and the salmon contributes omega-3 fatty acids, which are known to have anti-inflammatory properties. Another option is a quinoa breakfast bowl filled with fresh veggies like cucumber, cherry tomatoes, and kale, drizzled with olive oil and lemon juice for extra flavor and antioxidants.

Try this tofu scramble seasoned with turmeric, garlic powder, and nutritional yeast for a high-protein, balanced breakfast. Tofu is a great source of calcium and protein from plants, so it's a great choice for supporting bone and muscle health.

Serve with a side of steamed greens or a slice of whole-grain toast. If you'd rather have something sweeter, try these delicious, high-protein, and high-fiber almond flour pancakes with mixed berries and Greek yogurt on top.

BREAKFASTS THAT HELP CONTROL SYMPTOMS OF LUPUS

Prepare turmeric-spiced oatmeal cooked in coconut milk and top with sliced bananas and hemp seeds for a warming option. Fight lupus symptoms with these breakfast ideas that are meant to promote overall wellness and reduce inflammation. Begin your day with a green tea smoothie infused with fresh ginger and a squeeze of lemon. Green tea is rich in antioxidants that help reduce inflammation, while ginger supports digestion and immune function. Pair with a small serving of nuts or seeds for added protein and healthy fats.

If you're in the mood for a refreshing start, blend up a citrus and beet smoothie packed with vitamin C and nitrates that help improve blood flow and support cardiovascular health. Add a scoop of protein powder or Greek yogurt for added protein and creaminess. Bake until golden brown and serve with a side of mixed greens dressed with olive oil and balsamic vinegar. Another healthy breakfast option is an omega-3 enriched spinach and mushroom frittata. Spinach provides vitamins A and C, essential for immune health, while the mushrooms add selenium and antioxidants. Bake until golden brown and serve with a side of mixed greens dressed with olive oil and balsamic vinegar.

NUMEROUS TASTES AND CHOICES

A tasty option for keeping your morning routine interesting is a Mexican-style breakfast burrito made with scrambled eggs, black beans, salsa, and toasted coconut flakes wrapped in a gluten-free tortilla. Black beans offer fiber and plant-based protein, while salsa adds a burst of flavor and antioxidants. Start with a tropical fruit parfait layered with coconut yogurt, mango chunks, and a sprinkle of toasted coconut flakes.

Coconut yogurt is dairy-free and rich in probiotics, supporting gut health and immune function.

Breakfast brochette with hummus, cherry tomatoes, and fresh basil on gluten-free bread is a Mediterranean-inspired dish that provides plant-based protein and fiber along with vitamins and minerals from the tomatoes and basil. If you'd rather go lighter, try a fruit and nut bowl with seasonal fruits like kiwi, berries, and pomegranate seeds, topped with walnuts or crushed almonds for crunch and omega-3 fatty acids. These dishes not only taste good but also provide vital nutrients that support your general health and well-being.

OPTIONS FOR A SATISFYING AND HEALTHFUL LUNCH

It's important to find a balanced lunch that includes a variety of lean proteins, whole grains, and plenty of vegetables if you want to stay energized throughout the day. Lunch ideas like quinoa salads with chickpeas and mixed greens are a great way to get a good balance of protein, fiber, and vitamins. Another great option is grilled chicken wraps with whole-wheat tortillas, which are loaded with veggies like spinach, tomatoes, and avocado for extra flavor and nutrition.

If you'd like to include more plant-based options, try making Buddha Bowls, which are made with brown rice or quinoa as the base and topped with a variety of roasted vegetables, hummus, and a drizzle of tahini dressing. These bowls are visually appealing and high in fiber and antioxidants. You can also go ahead and bring hearty soups, like minestrone or lentil soup, to work in a thermos, which will keep you full and satisfied on chilly days.

The secret to maintaining a healthy lunch routine is planning. Cooking in large quantities on the weekends can free up time during the hectic workweek, enabling you to quickly put together wholesome meals. By emphasizing whole foods and sensible portion sizes, you can make lunches that promote your general health and sustain your energy levels throughout the afternoon.

IDEAS FOR CONVENIENT LUNCHES AT WORK OR SCHOOL

Portability and convenience are key factors when packing lunches for work or school. Choose meals that are easy to carry and don't need to be reheated, like grain-based salads like couscous with roasted vegetables and feta cheese. These salads are not only delicious but also withstand well in lunch boxes or other containers, making them ideal for hectic days spent on the go.

Sandwiches and wraps make great lunch options as well. Start with whole-grain wraps or bread and stuff them with lean proteins like grilled chicken or turkey, lots of crisp lettuce, sliced cucumbers, and a smear of hummus or avocado for extra flavor and nutrition. These options are adaptable and can be made to your personal preferences.

Bento box-style lunches are a lighter option that features sections for each food group. Stuff your box with sliced fruits, nuts, whole-grain crackers, and a portion of protein like tofu cubes or hard-boiled eggs. This method guarantees a balanced meal and makes it simple to snack on throughout the day.

Lunch packing can be made more effective and eco-friendly by investing in high-quality lunch containers and reusable utensils. If you plan and select foods that travel well, you can have wholesome meals wherever your day takes you, without compromising taste or health benefits.

RECIPES BRIMMING WITH ANTI-INFLAMMATORY SUBSTANCES

Including anti-inflammatory ingredients in your lunch recipes can help with overall health and wellness, especially for people with conditions like lupus. To help reduce inflammation in the body, look for foods high in omega-3 fatty acids, like walnuts or salmon salad with mixed greens and a lemon-tahini dressing. This recipe combines healthy fats, protein, and leafy greens for a filling lunch.

Another powerful anti-inflammatory spice is turmeric, which can be added to curries or roasted vegetables. Its active ingredient, curcumin, has been demonstrated to possess strong antioxidant qualities, which makes it a useful addition to your lunchtime repertoire. For a tasty and health-promoting lunch option, try making lentil soup infused with turmeric or roasting cauliflower with turmeric and chickpeas.

Add a lean protein like grilled chicken or tofu to round out the meal and give you energy for the rest of the day. Leafy greens like kale, spinach, and Swiss chard are rich in vitamins, minerals, and phytonutrients that can help combat inflammation.

Make colorful salads with a mix of these greens, topped with colorful vegetables like bell peppers, cherry tomatoes, and shredded carrots.

It is possible to support your body's natural healing processes and promote overall well-being by focusing on whole, nutrient-dense foods and adding anti-inflammatory ingredients to your lunch recipes.

Try experimenting with different flavors and textures to make meals that are not only delicious but also helpful in managing inflammation.

LUNCHES TO INCREASE VITALITY

Lunches that increase energy are essential for sustaining focus and productivity throughout the day. Include complex carbohydrates, such as whole grains, in your meals for a consistent energy release. For a light and filling lunch, try quinoa bowls topped with black beans, corn, and avocado and seasoned with lime juice and cilantro.

Make these meals ahead of time and portion them out for easy grab-and-go lunches during busy weekdays. Protein-rich meals, like grilled chicken with quinoa and roasted vegetables, also help sustain energy levels. Protein helps stabilize blood sugar levels and keeps you feeling full longer, preventing mid-afternoon energy crashes.

Consuming foods high in water content, such as cucumber, celery, and citrus fruits, can also help you stay hydrated and sustain your energy levels throughout the day. For a healthy midday pick-me-up, try some fresh fruit or veggie sticks with hummus.

To avoid energy dips, steer clear of heavy, greasy foods and sugary snacks in favor of nutrient-dense meals that support overall well-being and provide sustained energy. Planning and making thoughtful choices allows you to enjoy lunches that fuel your body and mind, keeping you focused and alert all day.

Carefully planning and considering food choices and storage techniques are necessary when packing nutritious lunches. To ensure a balanced meal, start by selecting a variety of foods from different food groups, such as lean proteins like grilled chicken, tofu, or beans; whole grains like brown rice or whole-wheat pasta; and an abundance of colorful vegetables and fruits.

Organize and prevent sogginess by keeping different components of your meal separate and organized using compartmentalized bento boxes or stackable containers. Invest in high-quality, leak-proof, BPA-free, microwave-safe containers for easy reheating and storage.

Make big batches of grains, proteins, and roasted vegetables at the start of the week and put them together into meals as needed. This way, you can mix and match ingredients for variety and make sure you always have a healthy option available. Make lunches ahead of time to save time on hectic mornings.

Assist in preventing overeating later in the day by packing small portions of nuts or seeds separately to sprinkle over salads or yogurt for added crunch and flavor. Incorporate healthy fats such as avocado, nuts, or seeds into your lunches to help keep you full and satisfied.

With careful planning and preparation, packing nutritious lunches can be both convenient and enjoyable, ensuring you have the energy and nourishment you need to tackle your day. By implementing a variety of nutritious foods into your lunches, you can maintain a balanced diet and support your overall health and well-being.

SCRUMPTIOUS AND FILLING DINNER OPTIONS

Finding tasty and satisfying dinner options will turn your lupus diet into a delightful culinary adventure. Emphasize combining whole, fresh foods that are high in antioxidants and anti-inflammatory qualities, like leafy greens, colorful vegetables, lean proteins, and healthy fats. Start with colorful salads with a range of textures and flavors, topped with avocado, nuts, and berries for extra taste and nutrition.

Try grilled or roasted vegetables with herbs and spices to add flavor without too much salt or sugar. Add lean protein sources, like grilled chicken or fish seasoned with citrus and herbs, for a light but filling meal.

Use whole grains, like brown rice or quinoa, as the foundation for hearty bowls filled with vegetables and garnished with seeds or olive oil for extra crunch and nutrition.

A satisfying and warm dinner option would be to try soups and stews made with vegetables, legumes, and lean meats simmered in flavorful broths.

These meals are rich in nutrients that are necessary for maintaining general health and well-being, and because they are made with whole, nutrient-dense ingredients, you can make dinners that taste good and help manage lupus symptoms.

ONE-POT DINNERS FOR SIMPLE CLEANING

For people who are managing a lupus diet, one-pot meals are a lifesaver as they minimize cleanup while optimizing taste and nutrition. Consider options such as hearty vegetable stews, in which all ingredients simmer together, infusing flavors and nutrients into every spoonful. Use a variety of colorful vegetables, beans, and lean proteins such as chicken or tofu for a balanced meal.

For more fiber and long-lasting energy, try adding whole grains like barley or quinoa to one-pot meals.

Since these grains take flavors well, they work well in pilafs and grain-based salads. Try experimenting with different herbs and spices to bring out the flavor profile without using too much salt or bad fats.

One way to simplify your lupus diet without sacrificing taste or nutrition is to embrace one-pot meals. Slow cooker recipes, which turn simple ingredients into hearty, flavorful dinners with minimal effort, allow ingredients to meld together over hours of gentle cooking. From rich, vegetable-packed chilis to tender braised meats, the slow cooker can do it all.

RECIPES TO SUPPORT HEALTHY JOINTS

For those with lupus, maintaining joint health is essential, and some recipes can assist with this aspect of overall wellness. One way to support joint health is to incorporate foods high in omega-3 fatty acids, like salmon, walnuts, and flaxseeds, which have anti-inflammatory qualities that can benefit joint health. Try making grilled salmon with quinoa and roasted vegetables for a well-balanced, joint-friendly dinner.

Taste turmeric, which has anti-inflammatory qualities; try curries or golden milk soups. Turmeric is a great addition to a lupus diet because it relieves stiffness and pain in the joints. It's also a great idea to eat lots of leafy greens, like kale and spinach, which are full of vitamins and minerals that support healthy joints.

Stir-fries with colorful bell peppers and broccoli seasoned with ginger and garlic can benefit from the addition of flavor and joint-supporting benefits from the inclusion of lean proteins like chicken or tofu. By carefully selecting ingredients and cooking meals that focus on joint health, you can improve your lupus management efforts while savoring delicious, nourishing food.

DINNERS TO PROMOTE HEALTHY DIGESTIVE SYSTEM

Encouraging regularity and overall digestive function is crucial for people with lupus, and dinner choices can make a big difference in reaching this goal. Start with foods high in fiber, like beans, and lentils, and whole grains like brown rice or oats.

Build meals around these components, adding colorful veggies like bell peppers, carrots, and leafy greens for extra fiber and nutrients.

Try using probiotics-rich foods, such as yogurt or kefir, in marinades or dressings to improve flavor and support gut health. These foods are full of good bacteria that support a healthy digestive tract and can help reduce symptoms like bloating and discomfort. Fermented foods, such as kimchi or sauerkraut, can be added to dishes to further improve digestive wellness.

Prioritize foods that support digestive health so that you can enjoy satisfying dinners that also help manage your lupus symptoms. Steaming or poaching are two gentle cooking methods that help retain nutrients and facilitate easier digestion. Avoid heavy sauces or excessive spices that may cause digestive distress and instead opt for light, flavorful seasonings like fresh herbs, lemon juice, or a drizzle of olive oil.

Mealtime can be made easier and everyone can enjoy healthy, delicious meals together if you find family-friendly dinner ideas that also follow a lupus diet. For example, you can start with flexible options like salad nights or build-your-own taco nights, where family members can customize their meals with different toppings and ingredients.

For a balanced meal, serve lean protein options like grilled chicken or beans along with a colorful array of vegetables and whole grains.

Incorporate kid-friendly favorites like homemade pizza with a whole wheat crust and plenty of vegetable toppings, making it an enjoyable and healthy dinner option for everyone.

Try pasta dishes made with whole wheat or gluten-free pasta options, served with a homemade tomato sauce packed with vegetables and lean ground turkey or tofu for added protein.

Using ingredients like sweet potatoes, lean meats, and legumes to create dishes that are satisfying and appealing to all ages is a comforting twist on hearty soups or casseroles that can be prepared ahead of time and reheated for busy evenings. By involving the whole family in meal preparation and emphasizing nutritious, balanced ingredients, you can create dinners that support both lupus management and family bonding.

HEALTHY SNACKS TO FIGHT MIDDAY HUNGRY FEELINGS

Choosing healthy snacks is important when fighting midday hunger pangs while following a lupus-friendly diet. These snack should give you sustained energy without making you feel irritated. Greek yogurt with fresh berries and a dash of chia seeds is one such option; the yogurt provides probiotics for gut health, and the berries offer antioxidants.

Raw vegetables like carrots, cucumbers, and bell peppers are another excellent option; hummus is high in protein and fiber, which helps you feel fuller for longer, and the vegetables provide vital vitamins and minerals.

If you are in the mood for something crunchy, roasted chickpeas seasoned with herbs or spices are a great snack. Chickpeas are high in protein and fiber, which helps to keep blood sugar stable. A handful of mixed nuts, like walnuts and almonds, also provide healthy fats and proteins.

These options are great for lupus patients who need to sustain their energy levels throughout the day because they not only effectively curb hunger but also promote overall health and wellness.

GUILT-FREE SWEET TREATS

A lupus diet doesn't have to be destroyed by sweets. Choose foods that emphasize natural sweetness and are low in added sugars. For example, make banana oat cookies with mashed bananas, oats, and a little honey or maple syrup. These cookies are easy to make and satisfy your sweet tooth without sacrificing your health. Another delicious option is a berry smoothie with almond milk and a dash of vanilla extract. Berries are naturally sweet and full of antioxidants, and almond milk provides creaminess without requiring dairy.

Greek yogurt with honey and mixed berries makes a cool dessert that can be frozen and then thawed into a guilt-free, creamy Popsicle that is ideal for cooling off on hot days. Another healthy option is to make almond butter-dipped dark chocolate, which is rich in antioxidants and can be melted and drizzled over fresh fruit for a sophisticated dessert that fits well with a lupus diet.

FOODS THAT GIVE YOU ENERGY FOR A LONG TIME

For example, a whole-grain wrap with lean turkey or chicken and fresh vegetables is a balanced snack high in fiber and protein. The complex carbohydrates in the wrap provide long-lasting energy, and the protein helps maintain and repair muscles. Another option is a quinoa salad with diced vegetables, chickpeas, and a lemon vinaigrette dressing. Choosing snacks that provide sustained energy is crucial for managing lupus symptoms. Choose options that combine complex carbohydrates with proteins or healthy fats.

Smoothies made with spinach, avocado, banana, and almond milk are also great options. The banana adds natural sweetness and potassium, and the avocado offers healthy fats that help with satiety. The spinach is full of iron and vitamins. The energy balls are made of dates, nuts, and rolled oats, and they make a great onthe-go snack. The dates provide natural sugars for instant energy, and the nuts and oats add fiber and healthy fats that help sustain energy levels throughout the day.

DESSERTS YOU CAN EAT IF YOU HAVE LUPUS

Sweets can still be enjoyed on a lupus diet as long as you choose healthy options. A fruit salad with honey and mint leaves is refreshing and full of vitamins and antioxidants. Other satisfying dessert options include coconut chia pudding, which is made with coconut milk, chia seeds, and a hint of vanilla extract. Chia seeds are a good source of fiber and omega-3 fatty acids, and coconut milk adds richness without dairy.

A warm treat that is low in added sugars is baked apples stuffed with a mixture of oats, nuts, and cinnamon; apples are naturally sweet and high in dietary fiber, and the oats and nuts add crunch and protein. Alternatively, a rich and creamy dessert is avocado chocolate mousse, which is made from ripe avocados, cocoa powder, and a sweetener such as honey or agave syrup.

Avocados offer healthy fats and a smooth texture, making this dessert lupus-friendly and satisfying.

OPTIONS FOR HOMEMADE SNACKS

Making your snacks helps you be more aware of what's in your food, which makes following a lupus diet easier. One great option is making your trail mix with a variety of nuts, seeds, and dried fruits. Go for unsalted nuts like walnuts and almonds, and add seeds like sunflower or pumpkin seeds for extra nutrients. Dried fruits like cranberries or apricots add natural sweetness without added sugars.

Another great homemade snack idea is veggie sticks with guacamole or salsa. Guacamole, which is made with mashed avocado, lime juice, and diced tomatoes, is high in antioxidants and healthy fats.

Making roasted kale chips with olive oil and sea salt is a great way to satisfy your savory snack cravings. Kale is a nutrient-dense leafy green that is packed with vitamins and minerals, and roasting it brings out a crunchy texture. Moreover, homemade energy bars made with oats, nut butter, honey, and dried fruits are a great way to grab a healthy snack quickly. You can customize these bars with your favorite ingredients and can easily make them ahead of time for hectic days. By making these delicious snacks at home, you can support your health and effectively manage your lupus symptoms.

DRINKS THAT ARE HYDRATING FOR PEOPLE WITH LUPUS

Maintaining proper hydration is essential for managing the symptoms of lupus because dehydration can worsen joint pain and fatigue. Patients with lupus can benefit from hydrating drinks that are more than just plain water, such as nourishing options that replenish electrolytes and support overall health.

One such hydrating drink is coconut water, which is high in potassium and electrolytes and is great for preventing cramps in the muscles that are commonly associated with lupus. Herbal teas, such as chamomile or mint, offer calming hydration with additional anti-inflammatory properties that can help to reduce flare-ups and stress.

Cucumber-infused water is a great option as well because it is hydrating and contains a refreshing dose of vitamins and antioxidants. Its natural detoxifying qualities can help reduce inflammation and support kidney function, which is important for people with lupus. You can also add fresh fruit juices, like pineapple or watermelon, to your water to stay hydrated and boost immunity because they are high in vitamin C. You should drink these hydrating beverages throughout the day to stay well-hydrated and to support overall wellness in people with lupus symptoms.

ANTIOXIDANT-PACKED SMOOTHIES

A berry blast smoothie, made with antioxidant-rich berries like blueberries, strawberries, and raspberries, provides a flavorful mix that supports immune function and reduces inflammation associated with lupus. A handful of spinach or kale boosts the smoothie's antioxidant power while providing essential vitamins and minerals.

Antioxidants play a crucial role in managing lupus by reducing oxidative stress and inflammation. Smoothies packed with antioxidants offer a delicious and convenient way to incorporate these protective compounds into your diet.

Green tea smoothies are also beneficial because they contain potent antioxidants called catechins, which have anti-inflammatory effects and may help manage lupus symptoms. Mango, pineapple, and kiwi are great fruit combinations for a tropical antioxidant smoothie. These fruits are packed with vitamin C and other antioxidants, helping to strengthen the immune system and protect against cell damage. For a creamy texture and added health benefits, consider using almond milk or Greek yogurt as a base.

Enjoy these antioxidant-packed smoothies regularly as part of a balanced diet to promote overall wellness and effectively manage symptoms of lupus. To maximize the antioxidant content, consider adding a tablespoon of flaxseed or chia seeds to your smoothies.

These seeds are rich in omega-3 fatty acids, which have anti-inflammatory properties and can further support heart health, a common concern for patients with lupus.

For those who have lupus, preserving gut health is crucial because gut health affects immune function and general well-being. Drinks that support gut health concentrate on boosting a healthy microbiome and decreasing inflammation.

One popular option for promoting gut health is kombucha, a probiotics-rich fermented tea that is rich in beneficial bacteria that support immune system function and digestive health. Regular consumption of kombucha can also help alleviate gastrointestinal problems that are frequently linked to lupus, such as bloating and irregularity.

Ginger tea is well known for its anti-inflammatory qualities and capacity to ease digestive discomfort. Ginger's natural compounds can help alleviate nausea and improve digestion, making it a comforting and therapeutic choice for lupus patients. Bone broth is another advantageous beverage, recognized for its gut-healing properties due to its high collagen content.

Collagen helps repair the intestinal lining and reduce inflammation, promoting gut integrity and absorption of nutrients crucial for managing lupus symptoms.

Drinks high in probiotics, such as kefir or yogurt smoothies, can also help support gut health by restoring good bacteria and facilitating better digestion. These tasty drinks offer a delicious way to improve nutrient absorption and maintain a balanced gut flora, which is important for immune system function and general health. By incorporating these gut-healthy drinks into your daily routine, you can improve digestive wellness and better manage lupus symptoms.

RECIPES FOR HERBAL TEAS THAT HELP RELAX

Since lupus patients often have disturbed sleep, chamomile tea is a popular choice for its gentle sedative effects and ability to promote sleep quality. Slurping up a warm cup of chamomile tea before bed can help soothe nerves, alleviate anxiety, and improve overall sleep patterns, contributing to better symptom management.

Herbal teas are well known for their calming properties, making them ideal for reducing stress and promoting relaxation, which is crucial for managing lupus symptoms.

Lemon balm tea is also beneficial for stress relief and mood enhancement, thanks to its natural compounds that support cognitive function and emotional well-being. Lavender tea is another excellent option, known for its relaxing aroma and calming effects on the nervous system.

This herbal tea not only promotes relaxation but also offers anti-inflammatory properties that can help reduce joint pain and inflammation associated with lupus.

By adding peppermint tea to your daily routine, you can create moments of calm and relaxation while supporting overall wellness and symptom management in lupus. Peppermint tea has cooling properties that provide relief from bloating and discomfort, making it a soothing choice after meals.

Peppermint tea also helps with digestion, which is something that lupus patients often experience.

Sustaining energy levels is critical for people with lupus because fatigue is a common symptom that can interfere with day-to-day activities. Boosting smoothie recipes aim to support immune function and reduce inflammation while offering sustained energy. One healthy option is a banana almond butter smoothie, which combines protein-rich almond butter and potassium-rich bananas for sustained energy and muscle support. Greek yogurt or almond milk is added for extra protein and probiotics, which support digestive health.

Adding a scoop of protein powder or a handful of nuts and seeds boosts the smoothie's nutrient content and gives you energy for the entire day. Citrus fruits like oranges or grapefruits can be added to smoothies for their vitamin C content, which supports immune function and enhances energy metabolism. A green power smoothie is another energizing option.

It features leafy greens like spinach or kale, which are rich in iron and vitamins essential for energy production.

Add a dash of cinnamon to your smoothies to further stabilize blood sugar levels and prevent energy crashes, promoting sustained energy and vitality. Turmeric's active compound, curcumin, has been shown to alleviate joint pain and inflammation associated with lupus. Ginger supports digestion and improves nutrient absorption. Turmeric and ginger smoothies are also beneficial for their anti-inflammatory qualities and ability to reduce fatigue.

You may effectively control your symptoms, boost your immune system, and fight exhaustion by including these energy-boosting smoothie recipes in your diet. This will enable you to live a more active and satisfying life while having lupus.

CHAPTER FIVE

PARTICULAR DAYS AND HOLIDAYS

ADVICE FOR MANAGING EVENTS AND GET-TOGETHERS

Managing a lupus diet at parties and get-togethers means being prepared and thoughtful. To start, let the host know what you need to eat so they know what to expect and can make accommodations. When you do go, make sure your plate is full of lupus-friendly foods like fresh veggies, lean proteins, and whole grains. Steer clear of processed foods, high sugar, and alcohol because they can aggravate your symptoms and cause inflammation.

When some foods are forbidden, it can be difficult to socialize. To ensure that you have something safe to eat, bring along a dish that fits your dietary restrictions and introduce others to tasty, healthful options. During the event, remember to stay hydrated and pay attention to your body's cues. Pace yourself, take breaks when necessary, and give priority to conversations over food so that you can fully enjoy the social experience without feeling deprived.

Remind yourself to enjoy the experience of interacting with others more than just the food. If needed, take up games or activities to take your mind off eating. If you are proactive and thoughtful, you can attend parties and get-togethers with grace and dignity while putting your health and well-being first.

RECIPES FOR THE HOLIDAYS THAT WON'T SET YOU OFF

Finding delicious, nutritious, and healthy holiday recipes for your lupus is essential to staying well. Try dishes like roasted veggies with herbs, grilled lean meats, or seafood high in omega-3 fatty acids.

Steer clear of flare-up-inducing foods like tomatoes and peppers, nightshade vegetables, and large amounts of red meat in favor of turkey breast, quinoa salads, or sweet potato mash seasoned with anti-inflammatory spices like turmeric and ginger.

Try desserts that are made without refined sugar, like honey or stevia. Fruit-based desserts, like baked apples or berry compotes, can satisfy a sweet tooth without sacrificing health. Try baking with gluten-free flour to make treats like coconut flour brownies or almond flour cookies, which can be enjoyed guilt-free during the holidays.

Make a plan and cook ahead of time using recipes that suit your dietary requirements. This will help you relax during the festivities and guarantee that you have nourishing options on hand. You can still enjoy holiday meals without sacrificing flavor or jeopardizing your health by using wholesome ingredients and being aware of potential triggers.

MENUS FOR SPECIAL EVENTS THAT PROMOTE WELL-BEING

Strategic planning and careful selection of ingredients are key to creating special occasion menus that promote wellness while managing lupus. Begin with balanced meals that feature a range of vibrant fruits and vegetables, lean proteins, and healthy fats. Add whole grains, such as brown rice or quinoa, for sustained energy and fiber. Steer clear of processed foods, high sodium, and saturated fats, as these can aggravate inflammation and aggravate symptoms.

Eat foods high in antioxidants and anti-inflammatory qualities, like grilled salmon with a citrus salsa or a vibrant salad with mixed greens, berries, and nuts. Add a lot of herbs and spices to boost flavor without using a lot of sauces or dressings. Drink hydrating drinks, like cucumber and mint-infused water, or herbal teas that aid in digestion and relaxation.

To make sure your menu selections for special occasions are in line with your health and dietary goals, seek advice from a nutritionist or dietician. By emphasizing nutrient-dense ingredients and thoughtful preparation methods, you can design menus that will not only promote wellness but also make your guests feel happy and fulfilled with delicious food.

FESTIVE SWEETS WITHOUT ENDANGERING HEALTH

A lupus-friendly diet requires creativity and mindfulness when selecting health-promoting treats for special occasions. Begin by looking into dessert options that substitute natural sweeteners like dates, coconut sugar, or fruit purees for refined sugars. You may also want to look into recipes for gluten-free cakes or muffins that use oats or almond flour as a healthy substitute for traditional baked goods.

Serve fruit skewers with a yogurt or nut-based dip for a cool and satisfying dessert option. For decadent treats, try making chocolate mousse with avocado or coconut milk, which has a creamy texture without the inflammatory effects of dairy. Add antioxidant-rich ingredients like dark chocolate, berries, or nuts to enhance flavor and nutritional value.

Planning celebratory treats should focus on moderation and portion control to prevent overindulgence. Provide a range of options to accommodate various dietary preferences and restrictions so that everyone can indulge guilt-free. that satisfy cravings and promote overall wellness.

To make sure you have options that support your health needs when attending social events, it's important to plan. Start by looking up the event location or getting in touch with the host to find out about menu options and accommodations for dietary restrictions. Be sure to express your needs clearly and courteously, making sure to emphasize your health concerns to ensure they are taken into consideration.

Plan for social gatherings by bringing snacks or small meals that fit your lupus-friendly diet. You can bring trail mix with nuts and seeds, fresh fruit, or make your energy bars with oats and dried fruit. This way, you'll always have a healthy option on hand in case there aren't many good food options available at the event.

CHAPTER SIX

CONTROLLING THE SYMPTOMS OF LUPUS WITH DIET

HOW INFLAMMATION CAN BE REDUCED BY DIET

Incorporating anti-inflammatory foods while minimizing those that can trigger inflammation is key to effectively managing lupus symptoms. Foods high in omega-3 fatty acids, like fatty fish (salmon, sardines) and flaxseeds, help reduce inflammation by inhibiting the production of inflammatory molecules. Other foods that help reduce inflammation include plenty of fruits and vegetables, especially those high in antioxidants, like berries and leafy greens, which help combat oxidative stress, which is a contributing factor to inflammation in lupus.

Processed foods and high sugar content should also be avoided as they can exacerbate inflammation. Instead, whole grains such as quinoa and brown rice offer nutrients and fiber without raising blood sugar levels.

Turmeric and ginger are natural anti-inflammatory spices that can be added to regular cooking to improve flavor and health benefits. People with lupus can better control their symptoms by emphasizing a diet high in anti-inflammatory foods and low in pro-inflammatory ones.

FOODS TO HELP WITH FATIGUE MANAGEMENT

Lupus patients frequently experience fatigue, and diet is a major factor in controlling energy levels. Eating small, frequent meals throughout the day helps prevent energy crashes and maintain steady blood sugar levels. Lean proteins like turkey, chicken, and tofu help maintain muscle mass and energy production. Complex carbohydrates like whole grains and legumes provide sustained energy.

Iron-rich foods (lean red meat, spinach, beans) should be included to help fight the fatigue brought on by anemia, a common lupus complication; vitamin B12, which can be found in foods like dairy, fish, and eggs, is also important for energy metabolism and nerve function; and drinking plenty of water and avoiding alcohol and caffeine can help prevent dehydration, which can worsen fatigue.

Individuals with lupus can better manage their energy levels and enhance their quality of life by focusing on nutrient-dense foods and maintaining a balanced diet. Meals should be balanced with a variety of nutrients to ensure that the body receives the necessary fuel to combat fatigue and support overall well-being.

BOOSTING BONE HEALTH WITH DIET

For people with lupus, who may be more susceptible to osteoporosis as a result of medication side effects and reduced physical activity, maintaining strong bones is critical. Calcium is found in dairy products like milk, yogurt, and cheese, as well as in fortified plant-based substitutes like almond milk and tofu. Vitamin D, which aids in the body's absorption of calcium, is acquired from sunshine exposure and foods like fatty fish (salmon, mackerel) and fortified cereals.

Additionally, foods high in magnesium and vitamin K, such as nuts, seeds, leafy greens, and cruciferous vegetables, can help support bone health. Merely including these nutrients in meals guarantees complete bone support. Limiting the intake of salt and caffeine is helpful because these substances can increase the body's excretion of calcium. By concentrating on a diet high in calcium, vitamin D, magnesium, and vitamin K, people with lupus can support bone health and lower their risk of fractures and osteoporosis.

DIETARY ADVICE FOR BEAUTY AND HAIR

Eating foods high in antioxidants, like berries, nuts, and green tea, helps protect skin cells from oxidative damage and promotes overall skin health. Omega-3 fatty acids, found in fish, flaxseeds, and walnuts, help maintain skin moisture and elasticity, reducing dryness and irritation. People with lupus often experience skin rashes and hair loss.

Vitamin E, which is found in nuts, seeds, and vegetable oils, also supports skin health by protecting against UV damage and promoting skin regeneration. Drinking plenty of water throughout the day helps keep skin hydrated and flushes out toxins that can contribute to skin problems. Eating foods high in vitamin C, such as citrus fruits, strawberries, and bell peppers, promotes collagen production, which is essential for skin structure and wound healing.

Protein-rich foods like beans, lean meats, and eggs support hair growth and strength. Biotin, which is present in eggs, nuts, and whole grains, promotes hair health and may lessen hair thinning. People with lupus can still have healthy skin and hair by focusing on a diet high in antioxidants, omega-3 fatty acids, vitamins C and E, and water.

METHODS FOR HANDLING WEIGHT WHEN LIVING WITH LUPUS

It can be difficult for people with lupus to maintain a healthy weight because of the side effects of their medications and their decreased levels of physical activity.

A balanced diet consisting of lean proteins, whole grains, fruits, and vegetables, as well as sugary snacks and processed foods, can help prevent needless weight gain and stabilize blood sugar levels.

Monitoring portion sizes and using mindful eating techniques, like chewing slowly and savoring each bite, can prevent overeating and support weight loss goals. Regular physical activity, like walking, swimming, or yoga, helps maintain muscle mass and promotes weight management.

Individuals with lupus can effectively manage their weight and improve overall health and well-being by adhering to a balanced diet, maintaining physical activity, and practicing mindful eating habits. Speaking with a registered dietitian can offer personalized guidance on nutrition and weight management strategies catered to individual needs and health goals.

CHAPTER SEVEN

HANDLING ALLERGIES AND DIETARY RESTRICTIONS

The first step in effectively managing lupus through diet is identifying foods that cause allergies or sensitivities. Common allergens like dairy, nuts, gluten, and shellfish should be avoided if they cause negative reactions. A registered dietitian or healthcare provider can assist in creating a customized meal plan that eliminates these allergens while maintaining a balanced diet. You can incorporate substitutions like almond milk for dairy or gluten-free grains to keep your diet interesting and nutrient-dense.

Apart from allergies, take into account dietary restrictions that could affect how your lupus is managed. For example, some lupus patients find that cutting back on red meat or processed foods helps reduce symptoms like fatigue and inflammation. Try different plant-based proteins like tofu, lentils, and beans to meet your protein needs while lowering the likelihood of triggers. Read food labels carefully to make sure you don't have any hidden allergies or ingredients that could aggravate symptoms.

To ensure that your meals are in line with your dietary restrictions and promote overall health by minimizing processed foods and additives, plan your meals and make homemade dishes whenever you can. By proactively addressing dietary restrictions and allergies, you can optimize your diet to support lupus management effectively.

MANAGING FOOD AND MEDICATION INTERACTIONS

To ensure optimal effectiveness and safety, people with lupus need to navigate the food interactions associated with certain medications. For example, certain medications may negatively interact with grapefruit or leafy greens, affecting absorption or increasing side effects. It is important to discuss these interactions with your healthcare provider or pharmacist to know which foods to avoid or limit while taking your medications.

Understanding these guidelines helps maintain consistency in medication effectiveness and lowers the risk of side effects. Some medications may require taking on an empty stomach, while others may be better absorbed with food. To manage medication interactions effectively, think about timing your meals around medication doses as advised by your healthcare provider.

To ensure that you can enjoy a varied diet while managing your lupus effectively, keep a list of all of your medications along with their specific dietary requirements close at hand. If you have any concerns about particular food interactions, speak with your healthcare team for individualized advice specific to your medication regimen and dietary requirements.

HOW TO EAT OUT WHILE HAVING LUPUS

When dining out with lupus, it's important to plan to maintain a healthy diet while managing symptoms. Look for restaurants that have menu items that fit your dietary requirements and preferences; many now provide information about allergens and healthier options, so it's easier to find options that work for you. When making reservations, let the staff know about any dietary needs or allergies to ensure a seamless dining experience.

If you have any concerns about a menu item, don't be afraid to ask questions about the preparation methods or ingredients used. If possible, choose dishes that are grilled, steamed, or baked rather than fried or heavily sauced.

This flexibility allows you to request modifications such as changing the ingredients or the seasoning to accommodate your health needs.

Planning and communicating your needs can make dining out with lupus enjoyable while supporting your health goals. Take your time perusing the menu and don't feel rushed into making a decision. Concentrate on choosing nutrient-rich options that include lean proteins, whole grains, and plenty of vegetables.

Bringing along snacks or small portions of safe foods can also provide backup in case suitable options are limited.

KNOWING INGREDIENTS AND LABELS ON FOOD

For people with lupus, reading food labels is crucial to avoiding triggers and ensuring adequate nutrition. Look for common allergens or additives that could aggravate symptoms in the ingredient list; ingredients like artificial preservatives, flavor enhancers, and high sodium content can cause inflammation and should be reduced or avoided.

Look for products labeled as organic or natural, as they often contain fewer additives and are less likely to cause adverse reactions. Become familiar with terms like "gluten-free," "dairy-free," or "low sodium" to identify products that align with your dietary preferences and restrictions. Pay attention to serving sizes and nutrient content per serving to make informed decisions about portion sizes and overall nutritional intake.

Fresh, whole foods are less likely to have allergens or hidden ingredients, so include them in your diet whenever you can. Lean proteins and produce from your local area will help you consume more nutrients and reduce your exposure to potentially harmful additives. Once you are proficient at reading food labels, you will be able to make confident food choices that will support your overall health and well-being while managing your lupus.

RESPONSES TO COMMONLY ASKED QUESTIONS

Here are some answers to some of the most common questions regarding food choices and how they affect symptoms when navigating a lupus diet.

1. Can some foods make lupus symptoms worse? Although everyone reacts differently, some lupus patients find that foods high in sugar, sodium, or saturated fats can make symptoms like fatigue and inflammation worse. It's important to keep an eye on how your body reacts to different foods and modify your diet accordingly.

2. Incorporating a range of fruits, vegetables, whole grains, and lean proteins into your diet can support overall health and potentially reduce inflammation associated with lupus; omega-3 fatty acids found in fish like salmon and flaxseeds may also have anti-inflammatory properties. Are there specific foods that can help manage lupus symptoms?

3. How should I handle alcohol consumption with lupus? Before consuming alcohol, it's best to speak with your healthcare provider about safe limits and potential interactions. Alcohol can exacerbate symptoms in certain lupus patients and interact with medications.

4. Is it wise for me to consider using dietary supplements to treat my lupus? While some people may find that taking supplements helps them, it's best to discuss their use with your doctor. Certain supplements, such as omega-3 fatty acids and vitamin D, may enhance overall health, but dose and medication interactions must be carefully taken into account.

5. How can I manage dietary restrictions and yet have a balanced diet? A licensed dietitian may provide direction, as can meal planning, to ensure that your diet is nutritious and balanced while taking into account any dietary restrictions or allergies. To make your meals pleasurable and fulfilling, try experimenting with different recipes and concentrate on complete, nutrient-dense foods.

People with lupus can improve their nutrition and successfully manage their condition by implementing tailored dietary methods and answering these commonly requested questions. A nutritious, well-balanced diet customized to each person's needs can be further supported by continuing self-monitoring and maintaining regular contact with healthcare specialists.